# Treat Your Own Hand and Thumb Osteoarthritis

*by*
*Jim Johnson, PT*

*This book was designed to provide accurate information in regard to the subject matter covered. It is sold with the understanding that the author is not engaged in rendering medical, psychological, or other professional services. If expert assistance is required, the services of a professional should be sought.*

Drawings by Eunice Johnson

Copyright © 2010, 2019 Jim Johnson

Published by Gatekeeper Press
2167 Stringtown Rd, Suite 109
Columbus, OH 43123-2989
www.GatekeeperPress.com

ISBN: 9781642376470
Library of Congress Control Number: Applied For

Printed in the United States of America

## Why Is The Print In This Book So Big?

People who read my books sometimes wonder why the print is so big in many of them. Some tend to think it's because I'm trying to make a little book bigger or a short book longer.

Actually, the main reason I use bigger print is for the same reason I intentionally write short books, usually under 100 pages–it's just plain easier to read and get the information quicker!

You see, the books I write address common, everyday problems that people of *all* ages have.  In other words, the "typical" reader of my books could be a teenager, a busy housewife, a CEO, a construction worker, or a retired senior citizen with poor eyesight.  Therefore, by writing books with larger print that are short and to the point, *everyone* can get the information quickly and with ease. After all, what good is a book full of useful information if nobody ever finishes it?

I have given my best effort to ensure that this book is entirely based upon scientific evidence and not on intuition, single case reports, opinions of authorities, anecdotal evidence, or unsystematic clinical observations. Where I do state my opinion in this book, it is directly stated as such.

—*Jim Johnson, P.T.*

# Contents

#  Hand Osteoarthritis: *Not* a Hopeless Case

**O**kay, you've got osteoarthritis in your hands. What now? We all know it won't magically disappear. Is it all downhill from here?

While these thoughts might have probably crossed some reader's minds, scientific studies that have followed people with hand arthritis for many years show us a much different picture. Consider this study published in the peer-reviewed journal *Osteoarthritis and Cartilage...*

- 59 subjects had X-rays taken of their hands (Harris 1994)
- 10 years later, they had X-rays taken again (their average age at this time was 69)
- 50% had worse hand arthritis
- 45% were unchanged
- 5% had *improved*

So if you thought hand arthritis only gets worse over time, the research shows us that this is not necessarily the case. In ten year's time, hand osteoarthritis hadn't progressed a bit in almost half of the subjects, and in fact, some people actually got better! This is encouraging, and now we know that if we have hand osteoarthritis, it's not necessarily an open and shut case that it will get worse over time.

However one thing we need to be aware of, is that X-ray studies like these only tell us what happens to *the structure* of your hand over time – not how your hand *feels* over time. Which brings me to another fact you may or may not know: *There is little association between how bad hand arthritis looks on an X-ray, and how bad it hurts.*

Here's what I mean…

- researchers studied 84 people who were *79 years old* (Bagge 1991)
- they also studied another 76 people who were *85 years old*
- X-rays were taken of their hands and graded from 0 to 4
- only 29% of subjects with grade 3 (moderate) and grade 4 (severe) hand osteoarthritis reported any complaints

It's quite noteworthy that these researchers found that 71% of subjects were walking around with grade 3 or 4 hand osteoarthritis (the worst kind) but had *no* pain. Along the same lines…

- a huge group of 1032 subjects, aged 71-100 years old, had their hands X-rayed (Zhang 2002)
- 89% of men had hand osteoarthritis, but only 9% of them reported any symptoms
- 94% of women had hand osteoarthritis, but only 17% reported any symptoms

So now you know that there can be little association between what a hand looks like on an X-ray picture, and how it feels.

Apparently a picture is *not* worth a thousand words, seeing as how it tells us little about how much pain an osteoarthritic hand has. So let's put aside the X-ray studies for now and check out one that looked at things from another angle, one that followed people with hand arthritis to see how their hands *felt and worked* over time…

- researchers followed 289 patients with hand osteoarthritis for 6 years (Bijsterbosch 2011)
- at the end of the study, 40% had more pain, 26% had less pain
- 50% ended up having a harder time using their hands, while 26% had an easier time using their hands

## So What's the Point?

While the studies we've just discussed might seem a bit boring, they do give the person with hand osteoarthritis a lot of helpful information. First of all, X-ray studies that follow people for *years* show us that the bones and joints of osteoarthritic hands do not necessarily deteriorate over time. In fact, half of the time, it's the case that people's hand bones and joints will either look the same *or* possibly improve over a ten-year period.

Secondly, don't let a bad X-ray report get you down either. Many studies have shown that there is little association between pain and how bad a hand looks on X-ray – and I have seen this many times over my 21 years as a physical therapist with other body parts such as the knee. Some people have lots of pain and very little arthritic changes in their hand – and vice versa. Keep X-ray results in perspective.

And perhaps most importantly of all, research shows us that it is *not* true that all osteoarthritic hands will continue to hurt more and more as time goes on. Recall the last study where over a quarter of people with hand osteoarthritis actually had *less* pain and an *easier* time using their hands as the years rolled on.

Having said that, however, we do have to keep in mind that there are also those with hand osteoarthritis that could have more pain and difficulty using their hands in the future. And, you probably are reading this book because you are having some problems with your hands already.

So to stack the odds in your favor, I'm going to show you things you can do, simple things, that will make your hands work and feel much better - now and over the long run – all proven to work in randomized controlled trials, the highest form of proof in medicine that a treatment is really effective. Specifically, in the pages to follow, you will find ways to effectively treat four of the biggest problems people with hand osteoarthritis have…

- hand pain
- hand stiffness
- decreased hand strength
- decreased hand coordination

So let's get started!

# Getting to Know Your Hand

**W**e've all heard the phrase "I know it like the back of my hand". Well, after this chapter, you're going to be a little more familiar with the front (and inside) too.

Why bother? Well, it's just going to be a whole lot easier getting your hand moving and feeling better when you know how it works. Let's begin with…

## The Bones

Now instead of just listing all the parts of your hand, and then giving you a boring medical definition, we're going to go over the hand's structures by taking a look at pictures of it from the *inside* out. Up first is the basic framework of your hand, *the bones…*

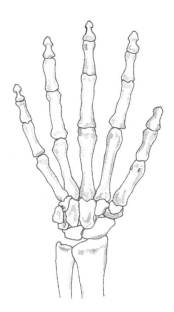

Figure 1. The many bones that make up your hand.

A look at Figure 1 quickly shows us that the hand is made up *a bunch* of bones. Here's a closer look at which ones make up your fingers, palm, and wrist…

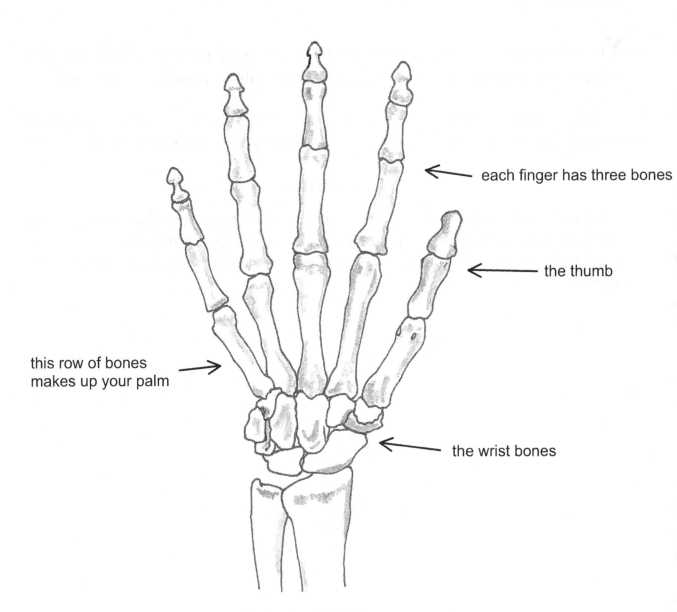

each finger has three bones

the thumb

this row of bones makes up your palm

the wrist bones

The right hand – palm is facing up.

And a more detailed picture of the many tiny bones that make up the wrist…

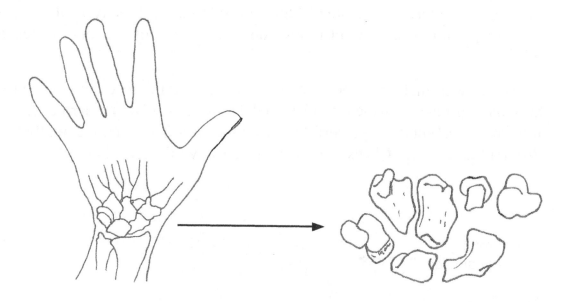

Figure 2. The right hand, palm up. Where the wrist bones sit.

Figure 3. What the wrist bones look like separated from each other.

## The Articular Cartilage

Now that you have an idea of what bones are in your hand, it's important to note that where they do come together and meet, their ends are coated with a substance called *articular cartilage*. Being very slick and smooth, it's a big job of the articular cartilage to decrease friction between the bones and help them move smoothly upon one another. Here's an example…

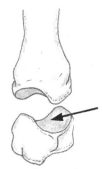

Figure 4. Arrow points to the articular catilage that coats the end of the bones.

Know that normal articular cartilage is a white, smooth, firm substance that is made up of cells called *chondrocytes*. However unlike other tissues in your body, like the skin or muscles, articular cartilage has *no* blood supply going to it. In other words, there are no small blood vessels going directly to it to provide life sustaining nutrients. So just how do these tiny little chondrocytes get their nutrition?

To answer that question, we have to take a microscopic look at how the articular cartilage is made up. If you take a piece of articular cartilage, and look at it from the *side* under a powerful microscope, you'd see that it actually has several different layers to it. Check out this picture and you'll see what I mean…

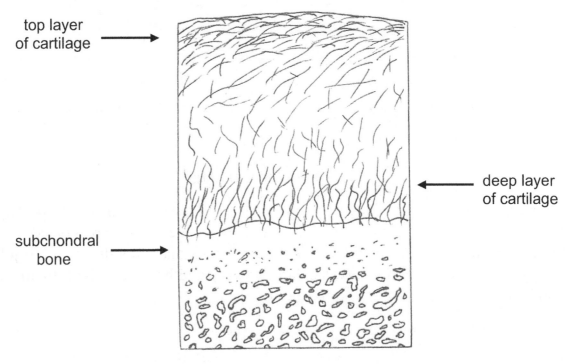

Figure 5. A sideview of the different layers of the articular cartilage. Note how the cartilage eventually blends with the underlying bone.

As you can easily see, there are several different layers to the articular cartilage. Scientists believe that the top layer gets its nutrition from a liquid floating around in the joints known as *synovial fluid*.

And the deeper layer of cartilage? It's most likely that it gets its nutrition from the *subchondral bone* it's right next to. In case you're confused, the subchondral bone is just a fancy name for the bone that sits *right under* the layers of cartilage.

### The Ligaments

Okay. Up to this point we've got an idea of what bones make up the hand, and we know that they are covered with smooth articular cartilage on their ends to help them glide easily on one another. So the next question is, what *keeps* the hand bones together? Well, it's a specialized connective tissue known as a *ligaments*.

Since it's the job of the ligaments to hold your bones together, it's logical that they'd have to run from one bone to another. Let's see what a few look like…

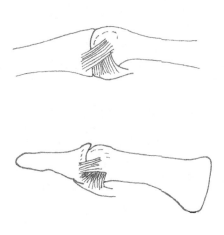

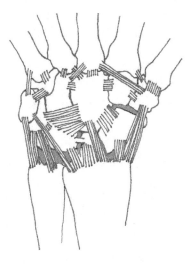

Figure 6. Ligaments holding the finger bones together.

Figure 7. The many small ligaments that hold the wrist bones together.

## The Synovial Membrane

I doubt a lot of readers have heard of this structure. The *synovial membrane* is like a "sleeve" that fits neatly around the joints in your hand and envelopes them. This is where it's located:

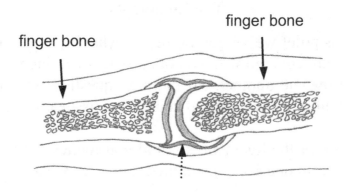

Figure 8. A finger joint. Dotted arrow pointing to the synovial membrane that is lining the inside of the joint.

Interesting structure, isn't it? Think of the synovial membrane kind of like a "plastic wrap" that clings closely to the entire finger joint.

So just what does the synovial membrane do? Well, it lines the joint and makes a substance called *synovial fluid*. Synovial fluid is a must-have for your finger joints because it floats around inside the joints, providing nutrients to the cartilage that coats the end of the bones. Additionally, it also helps lubricate your finger joints.

## The Muscles

We're finally to the last and one of the outermost structure of your hands - the muscles. On the next page is a look…

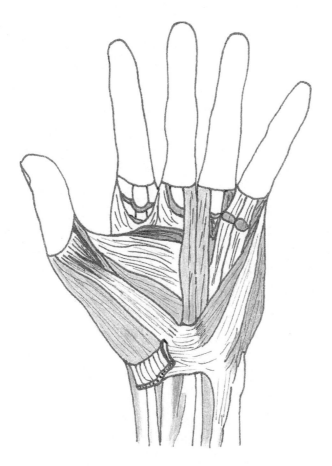

Figure 9. The muscles in the left hand – the palm is up.

As you can see, the hand is made up of *a lot* of tiny little muscles, each running in a slightly different direction. Of course it's the job of these muscles to move our fingers – which they do by contracting and pulling on the finger bones.

At this point, some readers might be wondering where the muscles in the fingers are? Well, there aren't any! Actually, the muscles that make the fingers move are located in your palm and forearm - and are connected to the fingers by long tendons.

Well, that's the basics. As we move through the rest of the book, we'll be referring to the hand's various parts from time – and now you know what they are and where they are!

# 3 **Getting Rid of That Stiffness**

If you're all too familiar with stiff hands and fingers that don't want to bend smoothly, you're going to like this chapter. Believe it or not, it is possible to decrease the stiffness and tightness that is so common in the wrist, hand, and fingers of osteoarthritis sufferers. So just how is that done?

By doing what are called *range of motion exercises* (or ROM for short). As a physical therapist, I use them all the time to restore the lost motion in joints. This type of exercise involves taking joints through their "range of motion", which stretches out tight tissues, makes the joints more flexible, and helps circulate the synovial fluid (page 10) that is so critical to joint health – which all helps to get rid of that "stiff" feeling in your fingers. But do they *really* help?

They sure do. Here's one such example...

- a group of patients with hand osteoarthritis were randomly assigned to a yoga program which included range of motion exercises, *or* to a control group that got no treatment (Garfinkel 1994)

- after 8-weeks, the yoga group significantly improved the flexibility of their hands compared to the control group

Know too that not only did the group that did range of motion exercises become more flexible and less stiff, but their pain levels and tenderness decreased as well! As you'll soon find out, range of motion exercises can be done practically anywhere and take only a few minutes each day to do...

Now before I show you how to do the range of motion exercises, I'm going to give you the option of applying heat to your hands to make the exercises easier to do. Heat makes molecules move faster, which means that heating the hand's tissues will increase your hand's circulation, makes the muscles and joints easier to stretch out, and besides all that – it just plain feels good!

If you have a heating pad, that's fine, use that. However if you don't, there is another, cheap way to go. In fact, all you'll need are three things:

A cotton tube sock…

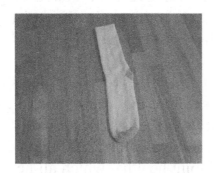

a bag of regular white rice…

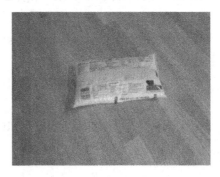

and a microwave…

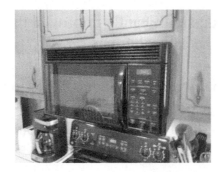

So here's what you do. Fill the cotton sock about ¾ of the way full of the rice. Make sure it's regular, uncooked white rice, and *not* instant or minute rice. This ordinary tube sock has been filled with a whole 2-pound bag of rice, but vary the amount as you see fit…

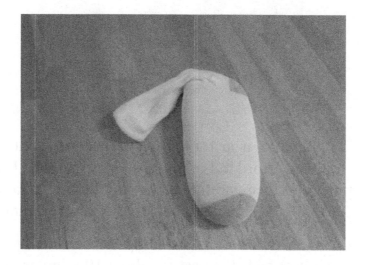

Next, tie off the top – it will look like this when you're finished…

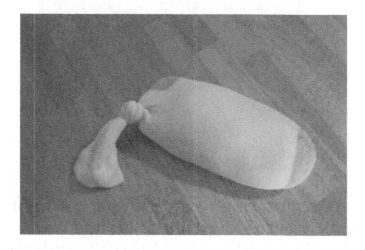

Now all you've got left to do is just pop it into the microwave and heat it up…

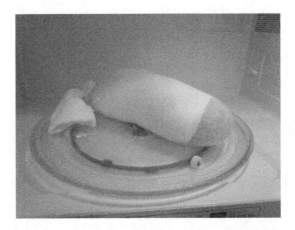

So how long do you stick it in for?  Well, that depends how hot you want it. It's going to be a trial and error kind of thing, so I recommend heating it up for one minute the first time, and then carefully checking the temperature to see if that's hot enough for your liking.  If not, put it back in for another minute and re-test.

Now when you have the rice sock heated up to your ideal temperature, just put the sock wherever the heat feels the best for about 10 minutes or so - whether it be on the top of your hand, the bottom of your hand, or sandwiched in between…

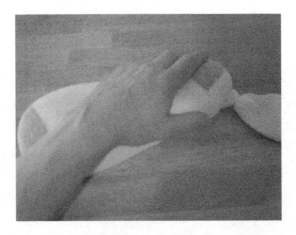

While applying heat to the hand is generally pretty safe for most people, there are certain medical conditions where feeling the heat can be a problem, such as with diabetic individuals – and one could possibly get burned.  This is why I recommend everyone check with their doctor before trying out the heated rice sock - just to make sure its okay.  Now on to the exercises…

## The Range of Motion (ROM) Exercises
## ROM Exercise #1

### Step One – start with your hand like this

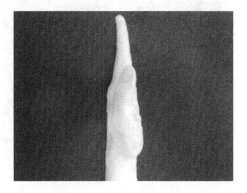

### Step Two – then bend keeping fingers straight

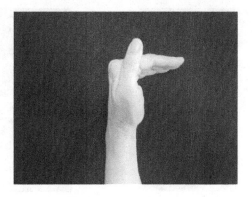

### Step Three – now return to the starting position
### and repeat 9 more times

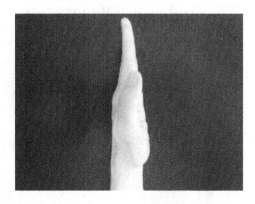

## ROM Exercise #2

### Step One – start with your hand like this

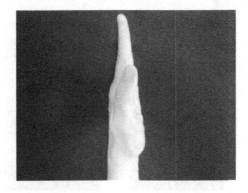

### Step Two – then bend fingers as shown in these side and front views

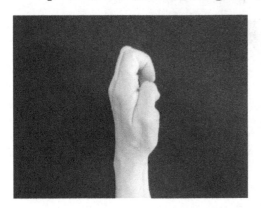 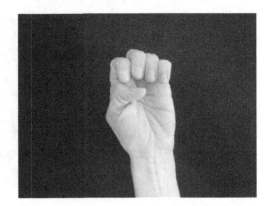

### Step Three – now return to the starting position and repeat 9 more times

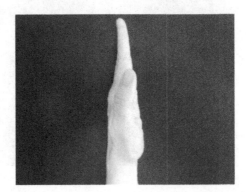

# ROM Exercise #3

## Step One – start with your hand like this

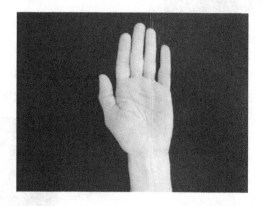

## Step Two – then make a fist

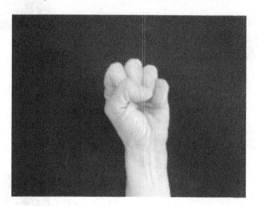

## Step Three – now return to the starting position and repeat 9 more times

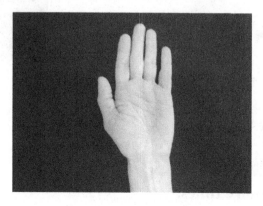

## ROM Exercise #4

**Step One – start with your hand like this**

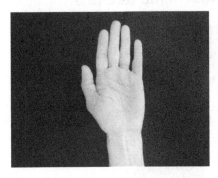

**Step Two – then make an "okay" sign with each finger**

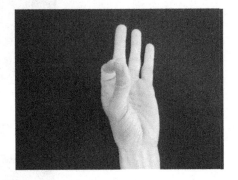

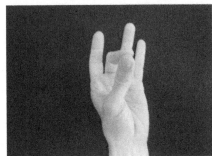

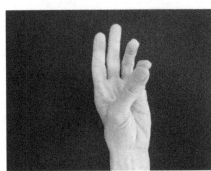

**Repeat 9 more times.**

## ROM Exercise #5

### Step One – start with your hand like this

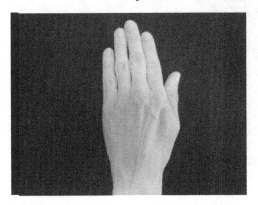

### Step Two – then spread your fingers far apart

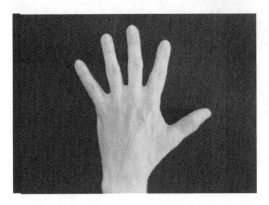

### Step Three – now return to the starting position and repeat 9 more times

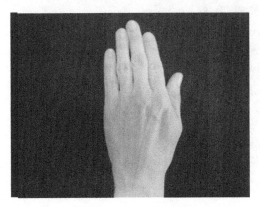

## ROM Exercise #6

**Step One – start with your hand like this**

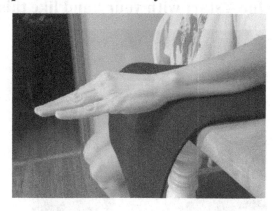

**Step Two – then, keeping hand straight, bend wrist *down***

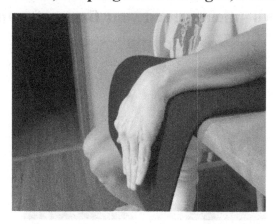

**Step Three – now bend wrist *up* while keeping fingers straight. Repeat this up and down motion 9 more times.**

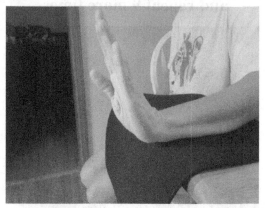

## ROM Exercise #7

**Step One – start with your hand like this**

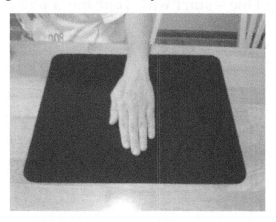

**Step Two – then, keeping the hand flat and fingers straight, rotate your wrist to the *left***

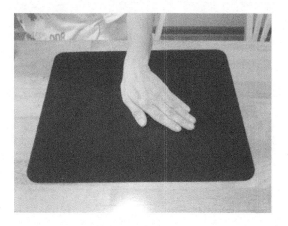

**Step Three – now bend the wrist to the *right* keeping hand flat and fingers straight. Repeat this left-right motion 9 more times.**

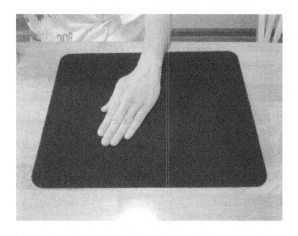

## ROM Exercise #8

**Step One – start with your hand like this**

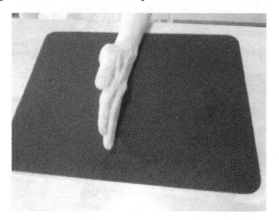

**Step Two – then, keeping your little finger in place, turn your palm *up***

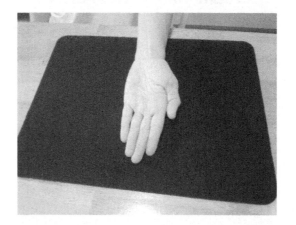

**Step Three – now, still keeping your little finger in place, turn your palm *down*.
Repeat this palm up/palm down motion 9 more times.**

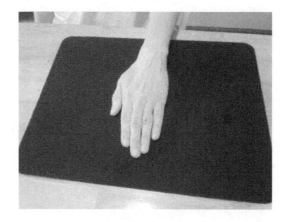

And there they are – eight range of motion exercises that stretch and lubricate every major joint in your hands to help eliminate stiffness. A few notes before beginning…

- *Where do I do them?* The ROM exercises can be done just about anywhere. For example, doing them on your lap while watching television is just fine - just make sure your hand is able to go through the correct motion of each exercise.

- *How often do I do them*? I recommend doing each exercise 10 times, one to two times a day – but they can be done any time your hands start to feel stiff.

- *Should I do them if I have pain?* Range of motion exercises help decrease pain, so it's okay to do them if you're having some pain. The key is to do them gently, BUT use common sense – if you're really having excruciating pain, or more pain than normal, you might be having a flare-up - and it's probably best to just let things rest until things settle down. As usual, check with your doctor before starting any new exercises.

- *What if my fingers can't quite get into the same position as in the pictures?* No problem – the key is to get as close as you can and work at it. In time, the joints and soft tissues in your hand will loosen up - and then you'll notice that you'll be getting closer to the positions in the pictures as time goes on. Once again, range of motion exercises are meant to be done *gently*.

# Making Your Hands *Stronger*

**D**o you feel like your hands are weaker than they used to be? Do you have trouble gripping or holding on to things? Well don't think things have to stay the way. I can name two, well done randomized controlled trials that have *proven* that people with hand osteoarthritis can make their hands much stronger in a matter of weeks...

---

### Study #1

- one randomized controlled trial tested 46 people with hand osteoarthritis (Rogers 2009)

- the control group used a fake hand lotion

- the other group did range of motion and strengthening exercises

- at the end of the study, the group that did strengthening exercises had improved their hand strength compared to the control group

### Study #2

- this randomized controlled trial involved 19 subjects with hand osteoarthritis (Lefler 2004)

- the treatment group did hand strengthening exercises

- the control group did nothing

- after 6-weeks, the group that did strengthening exercises improved hand strength significantly compared to the control group

---

And the good news is, it only took *a few* exercises for the people in these studies to increase their hand strength. On the next page are the strengthening exercises...

## Strengthening Exercise #1

**Step One – start out in this position using either no weight or a light dumbbell. You'll be sitting down with your hand hanging over the edge of a table**

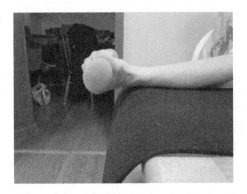

**Step Two – now smoothly bend your wrist *down*, letting the weight roll down your fingers an inch or two. If using no weight, just do the same motion.**

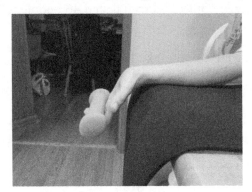

**Step Three – now curl your wrist *up*. And when you've curled it up as far as you comfortably can, I want you to hold and squeeze for a second or two at the top. Here again, if using no weight, just do the same motion.**
**Repeat this up/down motion 9 more times. When doing this 10 times in a row becomes easy, add more weight a pound or so at a time.**

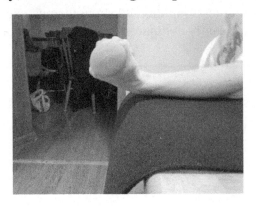

**Strengthening Exercise #2**

**Step One – start out in this position using a light weight. You'll be gripping the weight with *all five* of your fingers.**

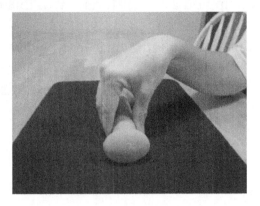

**Step Two – now smoothly pick the weight up off the table an inch or two - and hold for 3 seconds.**

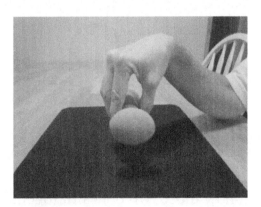

**Step Two – now put the weight back down on the table, rest for a second or two, and repeat 9 more times. When doing this 10 times in a row becomes easy, use a slightly heavier weight.**

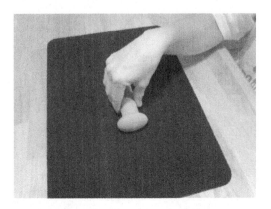

### And a Strengthening Exercise For Those With Thumb Osteoarthritis…

If you're having particular trouble with osteoarthritis of your thumb, I've got a strengthening exercise to help you out. Sufferers with this condition typically have pain at the bottom part of their thumb where it attaches to the palm, and over time, can notice the bones getting out of alignment. Here's what's going on…

A look at this picture shows us where the problems all start – at the bottom part of your thumb bone…

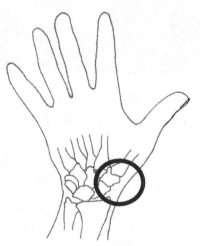

Figure 10. The right hand, palm up. Circle shows the two bones where thumb osteoarthritis commonly first starts.

And here's a closer look at how those two bones fit together…

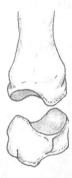

Figure 11. The joint at the base of your thumb.

Interesting little joint, isn't it?  It's got an interesting name too – *a saddle joint* – because it looks like a saddle of course.  And it's because of this odd shape that we're able to move our thumbs in a million different directions.

But that's just the problem.  Because our thumbs have soooo much motion in many different directions, it can overstress the delicate ligaments that hold this joint together.  Here's what the ligaments look like…

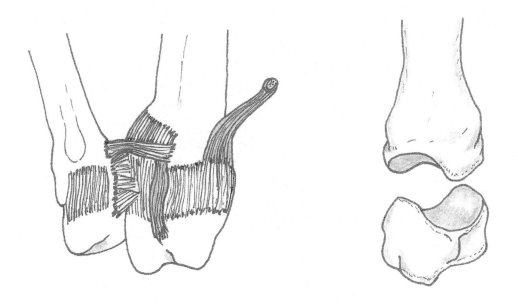

Figure 12. Left picture shows thumb joint with ligaments,
while the right picture shows joint without them.

Studies on people with thumb osteoarthritis have shown that over time, these ligaments can weaken, and in some cases, eventually become detached from the bone (Pellegrini 1991, Doerschuk 1999).  And when this happens, the bones aren't held together as tightly as they should - and the whole joint starts to become looser.  In time, the thumb bones can even shift out of place and stick out.

So what can be done?  Well, we know it's the job of the ligaments to hold the bones together and keep them in place.  So if your thumb joint is *losing* stability because of faulty ligaments, then we've got to find a way get some of it back to help keep the bones in place – but how?

Well, luckily you have *muscles*.  Along with making your bones move, the muscles also play a key role in *stabilizing* joints.  And one such muscle that is key in stabilizing your thumb, is the one known as *abductor pollicis longus*.  Let's take a look at it...

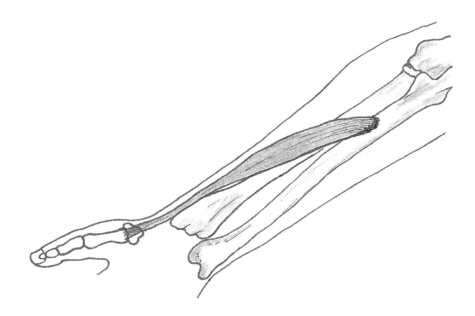

Figure 13. Looking at the right thumb and arm – the abductor pollicis muscle.

As you can see, one end of the muscle attaches in your forearm near your elbow, while the other end attaches to the thumb – right at that saddle joint where we need the most stability!  On the next page is an exercise to strengthen your abductor pollicis muscle to help stabilize your thumb joint...

## Strengthening Exercise #3

**Step One** – start out in this position. Your hand will be resting flat on a table. The thumb *must* be in line with your first finger.

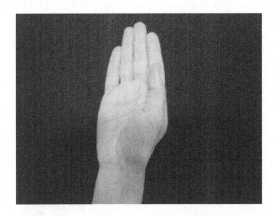

**Step Two** – now lift your thumb straight up, making sure to keep it in line with your first finger – as in these front and back views

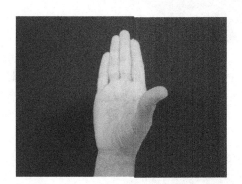 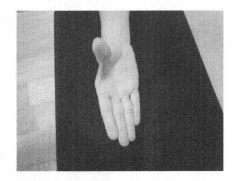

**Step Three** – now return to the starting position and repeat 9 more times

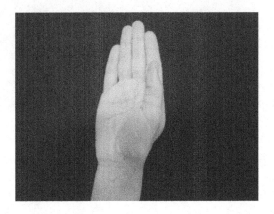

It's a simple exercise, but trust me, it works one of the most important muscles that helps stabilize your thumb joint (van Oudenaarde 1991, van Oudenaarde 1995).

One more thing, when you can do the exercise 10 times easily, you'll need to add some resistance to the thumb in order to keep getting the abductor pollicis muscle stronger. The simplest way is to use a rubber band. Here's what you do:

Buy a bag of rubber bands, they're cheap, and usually come in assorted sizes...

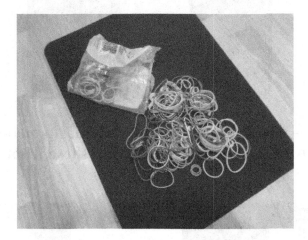

Find the thinnest one you can, like the one on the *right*, because it will be the easiest to start out with, unlike the one on the left...

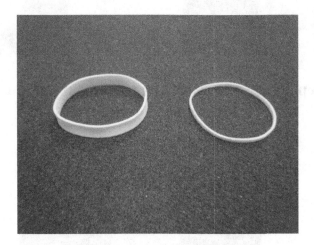

Next, place the rubber band around your hand like the picture below…

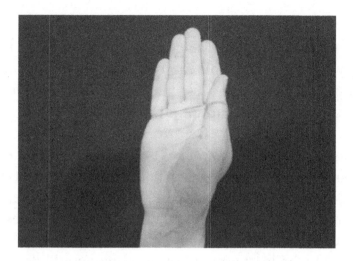

And then do the exercise as described earlier…

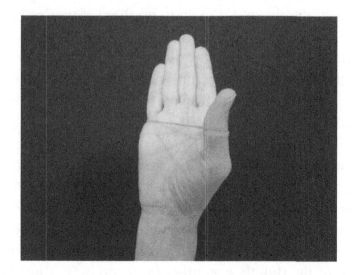

And that's it for hand strengthening!  A few notes before you jump in and start exercising…

- *Where can I do them?* The exercises can be done just about anywhere.  For example, doing them on your lap while watching television is just fine - just make sure your hand is able to go through the correct motion of each exercise.

- *How often should I do them?* I recommend doing each strengthening exercise once a day, no more than two to three times a week - with at least a day of rest in between exercise sessions.  For example, you could do them Monday, Wednesday, Friday, *or* you could do them Tuesday, Thursday, Saturday.  Twice a week is probably the least amount of times you could do them and still get stronger, so doing them on Monday and Friday would still work too.

- *Should I do them if I have pain?*  Strengthening exercises help decrease pain, so it's okay to do them if you're having some pain.  The key is to do them gently, BUT use common sense – if you're really having excruciating pain, or more pain than normal, you might be having a flare-up - and it's probably best to just let things rest until things settle down.  As usual, check with your doctor before starting any new exercises.

- *How much weight should I use?* It's okay to start out doing the exercises with no weight or a really light amount of weight – whatever your fingers will tolerate.  Then, when you can do an exercise 10 times easily – add a little bit more weight to challenge the muscle so it will get stronger (or a thicker rubber band in the case of the thumb strengthening exercise).  Repeat this process until you are feeling as strong and pain free as you want to be.

# Increasing the *Coordination* In Your Hands

**I**f you just can't seem to manipulate your hands like you used to and have trouble doing things such as writing, tying shoe laces, or fastening a button, then you're going to be happy you read this chapter. According to the latest research, we lose coordination in our hands as we get older - but that's a problem we can tackle…

- researchers tested 28 elderly subjects between the ages of 65 and 79 years of age (Ranganathan 2001)

- half were randomly assigned to a control group that did nothing

- the other half did an exercise to improve the ability to use their fingers better

- after 8-weeks, the exercise group were able to control their fingers better, had steadier hands, and much better finger coordination

Looks like all it takes is one simple exercise to work wonders for our hands *if* we know which one to do. But what one exercise could possibly do all that in a matter of weeks? Glad you asked…

### What You'll Need

The hand coordination exercise in the study involved subjects using two metal balls that were 2 inches in diameter…

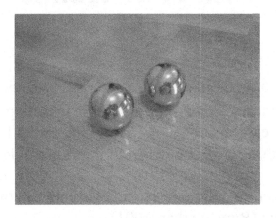

Do they have to be *exactly* 2 inches to get the same results? No. However if you try and use balls that are a lot bigger, you won't be able to do the exercise (because they have to both fit in your hand), and if you use balls that are really small, such as marbles, the exercise will be too hard to do – so try and get as close as you can to 2 inches. I obtained the above balls off the internet, and they cost around ten dollars. They're usually listed as "Chinese balls", "health balls", or "stress balls" – and are not at all hard to find.

So what exactly did the people in the study do with them? Well, it was a very simple exercise actually. All you do is take the two balls and hold them in the palm of your hand. Then, you practice rotating them *clockwise* for 10 minutes one time a day, and another 10-minute session later rotating them *counterclockwise*.

When I first learned about this study some time ago, I had my mother, who has hand osteoarthritis, try this exercise. She practiced with them twice a day, usually while watching television, and had great difficulty at first getting the balls to turn. After only a few weeks, however, she was amazed at how much easier she could manipulate them! On the next page are pictures of the exercise…

## Hand Coordination Exercise

**The goal is to rotate the balls in the palm of your hand for 10 minutes in a *clockwise* direction one session, and later, for 10 minutes in a *counterclockwise* direction. You may have to work up to the 10 minutes.**

**Follow the ball with the black square – in this example, it's being rotated *clockwise* …**

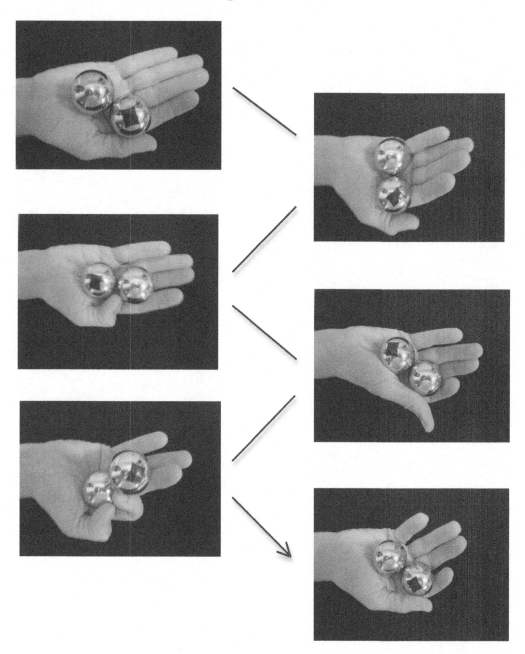

**…and you would continue this for 10 minutes.**

# How to Protect the Joints in Your Hand

If you're like most people with hand osteoarthritis, there are some activities you do that just don't agree with your hands – whether it's something as simple as opening a jar or twisting a key. And when you do one of these things, not only does it hurt, but the pain can sometimes last *long* after the activity is over.

Well that's a major goal of this chapter – showing you how to do the things you have to do *without* causing pain or injury to your hands. Physical and occupational therapists call it *joint protection*, and there's good research showing us that when joint protection principles are combined with other treatments, such as exercise or hand splints, patient's pain levels go down (Boustedt 2009) and hand function increases significantly (Stamm 2002).

---

**Take the Test!**

In the pages that follow, I'll be going over many, common, everyday activities that can put stress on an osteoarthritic hand and result in pain – and then I'll show you an alternative way to consider doing it.

After reading this chapter, you can prove to yourself just how quickly these minor adjustments can change your pain by taking this simple test.

Pick an activity that causes you pain, perform the activity, and then rate how much pain you have on a scale of 0 to 10 (0 is if you're having no pain, 10 is if you're having the worst possible pain).

Next, try doing the same activity again using the joint protection principles you've just learned in this chapter - and then re-rate your pain. The reduction in pain can often be quite dramatic! Case in point, all the pictures you're about to see (and in this book) were drawn by my mother who has hand osteoarthritis – which was only made possible by adapting her drawing instruments…

---

Instead of gripping a cup tightly by its small handle...

Try a mug and wrap your whole hand around it.

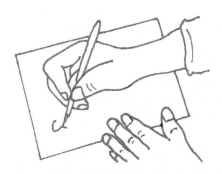 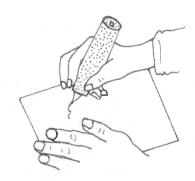

Instead of using regular pens and pencils...

Try building them up with foam, making them easier to hold.

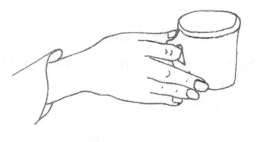 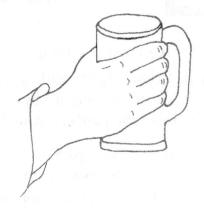

Instead of using these kind of faucet handles...

Try this kind where you can use the palm of your hand.

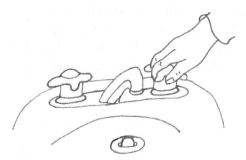 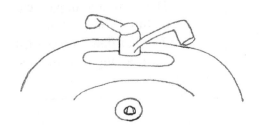

**Instead of pinching keys tightly to open things...**

**Try a key turner with a large handle.**

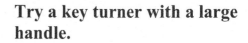

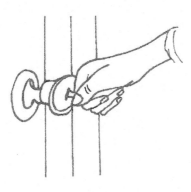
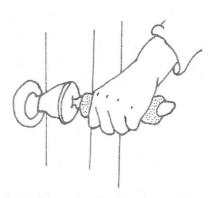

**Instead of using tools and equipment with narrow handgrips...**

**Try building up handles with foam or thick tape.**

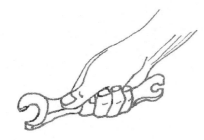
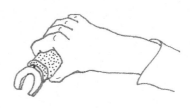

**Instead of using regular scissors...**

**Try using scissors with special handles.**

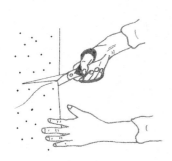
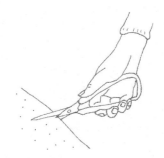

**Instead of using a regular can opener...**

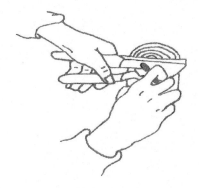

**Try using an electric one.**

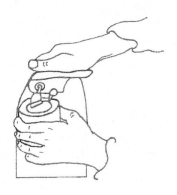

**Instead of opening jars by twisting with the fingers...**

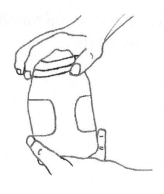

**Try using the palm of your hand instead.**

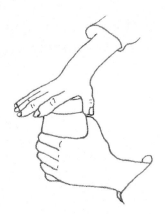

**Instead of stirring like this...**

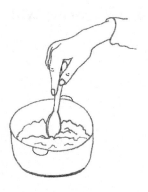

**Try stirring with this grip.**

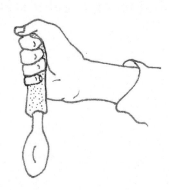

**Instead of using pans with one handle…**

**Try using pans with two handles whenever possible.**

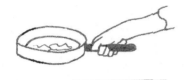 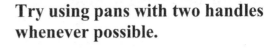

**Instead of using small handled knives and utensils…**

**Try using cutters, knives, and utensils with larger handles…**

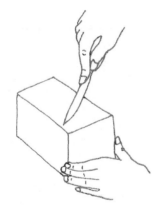 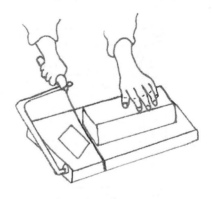

**Instead of wringing out cloths like this…**

**Try using a flat hand to squeeze the water out.**

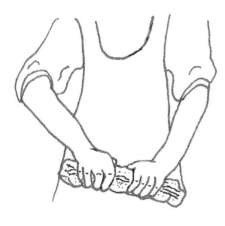 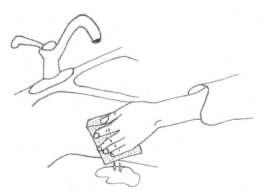

45

**Instead of wiping surfaces like this with a gripping motion...**

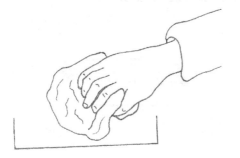

**Try keeping your hand flat to clean instead.**

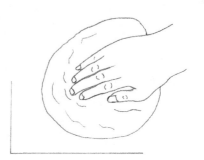

**Instead of twisting blinds open with your fingers...**

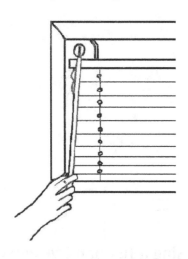

**Try building up the handles so you can use your whole hand.**

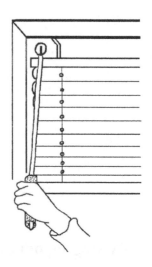

**Instead of using bottles that requires you to screw the caps on and off...**

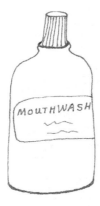

**Try pouring contents into bottles that you can pump with your palm.**

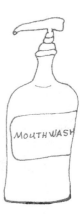

**Instead of squeezing tubes…**

**Try using many of the dispensers that are available.**

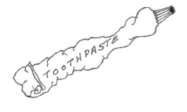

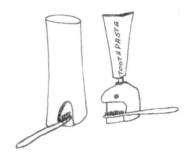

**Instead of carrying a purse in your hand…**

**Try carrying your purse on your shoulder or forearm.**

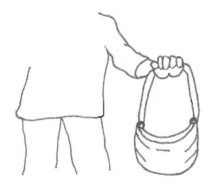

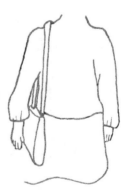

**Instead of lifting and carrying suitcases and bulky objects…**

**Try putting objects on wheels and pull them.**

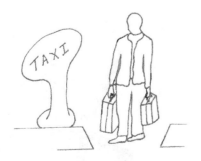

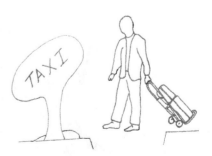

**Instead of resting your head on your knuckles...**

**Try resting your head on the heel of your hand.**

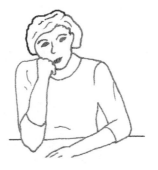 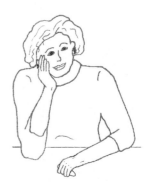

**Instead of using your fingers when getting out of a chair...**

**Try using the heel of your hand.**

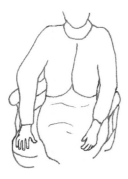 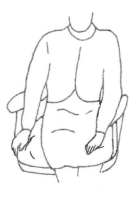

**Instead of gripping thin steering wheels tightly...**

**Try periodically relieving your grip and using padded covers.**

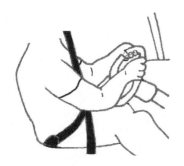 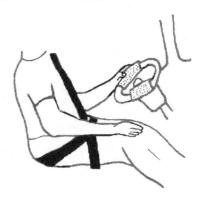

**Instead of holding the phone during long conversations...**

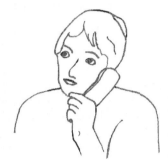

**Try using one of the many hands-free headsets available.**

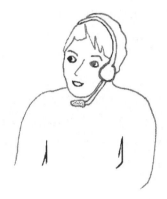

**Instead of using your fingers to help you carry objects...**

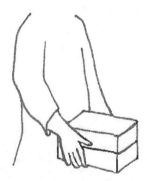

**Try using your forearms and keep things close to your body.**

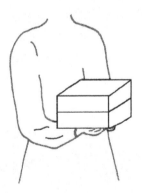

**Instead of pulling objects with your fingers...**

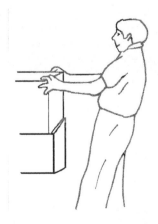

**Try pushing objects and using your bodyweight.**

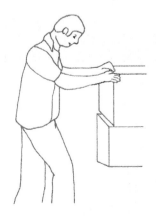

So what did you think?  Did you find any activities that cause you pain in particular?  I'm sure you found a few.  If you noticed, many of the alternatives involve changing the way you grip things.  Instead of using the small joints in the fingers and thumb (that are the weakest), the activity shifts to using the larger joints at the base of your fingers, palm, and wrist.

You also probably noticed that I mentioned several times to "build up" a handle or grip.  That's because small diameter handles and objects (like pens) require a much tighter grip to hold on to them – and a stronger grip means more stress on the joints in your hands.

On the other hand, a larger grip is much easier to hold to and you don't have to grip quite as tightly to hold on to things.  If you want to know a cheap, easy way to build up things like spoons, forks, pens, and other utensils and tools, a good way is to buy a tube of foam that is about an inch and a half in diameter with a hole in the middle.  Purchasing a couple of feet of this stuff, which is available at many hardware stores for example, allows you to cut off pieces to perfectly suit your needs.  Here are a couple of pictures of the stuff I use with patients…

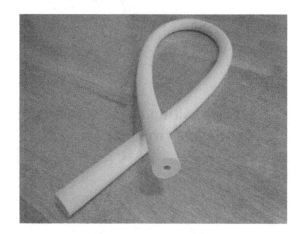 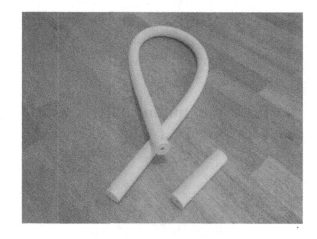

Yet other changes suggested involve using different utensils and equipment entirely to get the activity done safely – some you may have known about - while others you may not have.  If you look around at medical supply stores, or search the internet under "arthritis adaptive equipment", you'll find many more simple products that may be of great benefit to you, such as the following…

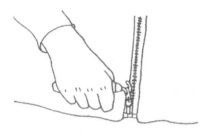

**zipper puller**

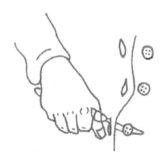

**buttonhook**

Well, that's it! It's time now to start thinking about the way you're using your hands throughout the day, pinpoint the activities that are creating stress and pain, and implement other ways of doing them. And remember, many times decreasing a lot of *little* stresses throughout the day can add up to *big* pain relief.

# 7  The Usefulness of Splints

A lot of people aren't crazy about wearing a splint on their hand. But before you rule one out, let me show you some pictures of the kinds of splints I'm suggesting you consider for your hand osteoarthritis – just so we're on the same page.

To begin with, the most researched splints for hand arthritis are the kind that are used for thumb arthritis. There are many types, but they basically look like this...

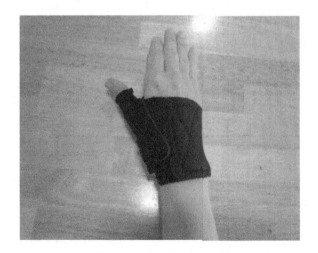 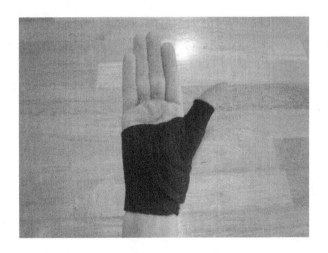

This particular kind is a soft splint that uses velcro to secure it. It's widely available on the internet, washable and allows you to use your fingers freely. Most readers know it "splints" the thumb, but let me tell you what all it can do for the person with thumb osteoarthritis...

They're pretty effective in decreasing pain…

---

- 40 patients with thumb arthritis were randomized into two groups (Carreira 2010)

- one group was instructed to wear a splint during the day

- the control group didn't wear a splint

- after 45 days, the splint group had a significant decrease in pain compared to the control group

---

Remember in Chapter 4 we talked about how in thumb osteoarthritis the whole thumb joint can become unstable because the ligaments weaken?  Well, when the thumb bones shift out of place, it's called a *subluxation*.  And according to studies, thumb splints can actually help *keep* the thumb bones where they're suppose to be…

---

- 25 patients were randomly assigned to wear one of two splints - one was a custom made plastic splint, the other a soft, prefabricated neoprene splint (Weiss 2004)

- subjects wore the splints whenever they felt symptoms

- after one week, patients rated their pain levels – and then each group switched splints for one more week

- at the end of the study, x-rays were taken to see how well the thumb bones stayed in place while subjects stressed their thumbs. Results showed that both splints stabilized the thumb joint and reduced subluxation.

- both splints were also effective in reducing pain

You can even wear them just at night if you want to - and they'll still work…

- 112 patients with thumb osteoarthritis were randomly assigned to wear a thumb splint, or no thumb splint (Rannou 2009).

- subjects who wore the splint, did so *only* at night

- one year follow-up showed that those who wore the splint had significantly improved pain and disability compared to the group that didn't wear the splint

And you don't even need a very fancy one…

- 10 subjects with thumb osteoarthritis tested out three different kinds of splints (Buurke 1999)

- one splint was made out of elastic, the other two were semi-rigid

- each subject wore each splint for 4 weeks in a randomized order

- at the end of the study, all three splints were found to decrease pain equally

As you can see, if you've got painful thumb osteoarthritis, a splint might be worth a try because…

- they've been proven to decrease pain

- they help even if you can wear them just during the day, or just during the night

- softer, more comfortable braces work just as well as plastic, rigid ones

- and x-rays have proven that even the soft splints reduce subluxation and keep the bones in place as you use your thumb!

So what about splints for the other fingers?  Well, they haven't been studied nearly as much as the thumb splints, but what studies have been done show they work pretty well.  For instance, a 2010 study published in the *Journal of Hand Surgery* showed that a tiny plastic splint reduced pain levels by 66% (Ikeda 2010).

They too are worth checking into, as they are cheap, lightweight, and easy to use.  Here's an example of a common plastic type, but many varieties are available on the internet…

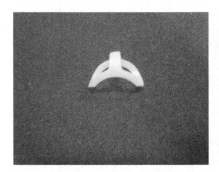 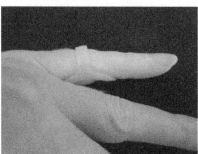 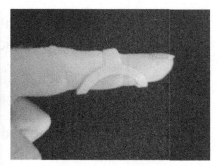

Splints – definitely worth considering!

# **8**   How to Stay on Track

Up to this point in the book, we've built a good foundation of knowledge for you to be able to treat your own hand osteoarthritis.  With that accomplished, it's now time to go over the six-week program I've laid out for you. Here are a few key rules to always keep in mind before you begin …

- always check with your doctor before beginning an exercise program. Physical and occupational therapists are always great resources as well.

- the number one rule is "Do no harm." You should not be in a lot of pain while doing these exercises. Some discomfort is okay, but remember that you're working muscles and joints you probably haven't used in a while, at least in this manner.

- stop the exercise if you have any significant increase in hand pain or symptoms. If done correctly, the exercises in this book do not stretch your hands in odd or unsafe positions, nor do they involve any heavy weights– and should be safe for your hands. *However*, they're your hands and your responsibility, so stop if you feel like any harm is being done.

# DO THESE EXERCISES ON MONDAY, WEDNESDAY, and FRIDAY

| These ROM Exercises Decrease *Stiffness* Do 10 times 1-2 times a day | These Exercises Increase Hand *Strength* Work up to 10 times in a row | This Exercise Increases Hand *Coordination* 1 Session - 10 mins clockwise 1 Session – 10 mins counterclockwise |
|---|---|---|

Page 17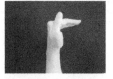

Page 28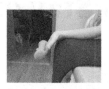

Page 39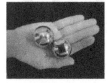

Page 18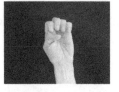

Page 29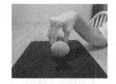

Page 19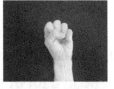

Page 33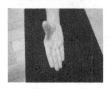

Page 20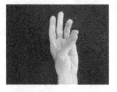

Page 21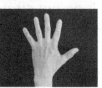

Page 22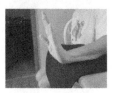

Page 23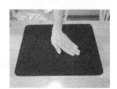

Page 24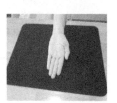

# DO THESE EXERCISES ON TUESDAY, and THURSDAY

**These ROM Exercises**
**Decrease *Stiffness***
Do 10 times 1-2
times a day
_____

**This Exercise**
**Increases Hand *Coordination***
1 Session - 10 mins clockwise
1 Session – 10 mins counterclockwise
_____

**Page 17**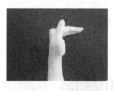

**Page 18**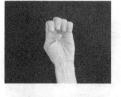

**Page 19**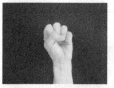

**Page 20**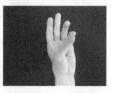

**Page 21**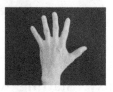

**Page 22**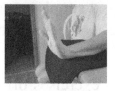

**Page 23**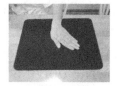

**Page 24**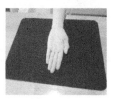

**Page 39**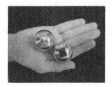

## Track Your Progress!

Since it can be hard to remember from one session to the next things like how much weight you used, it's helpful to quickly jot down this information. I've also found that when patients keep track of their exercises, it helps keep them on track too! The following is an example of how to record your progress by using the exercise sheets provided in this book…

### Week 3: Wednesday

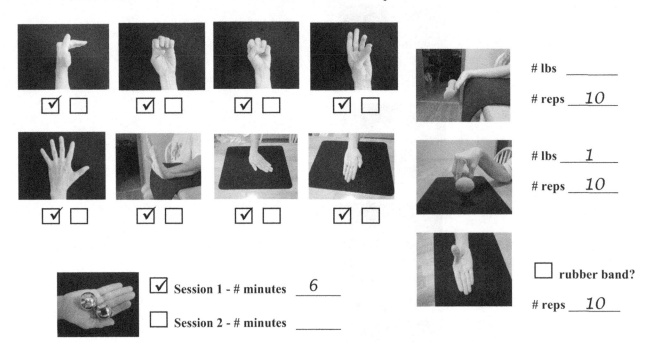

Using the exercise sheets provided is easy. Starting with the group of eight range of motion exercises in the upper left, you simply put a check in the box after you've done each one 10 times – there are two boxes, so shoot for doing them twice a day.

Next are the group of three strengthening exercises off to the right. You each one once a day – just fill in the amount of weight (if any is used) and the number of times (reps) you were able to do it on the lines provided. And last, down in the lower left, is the coordination exercise – shoot for doing that one twice a day for 10 minutes. If you can't do 10 minutes, simply write down how long were able to do it for in the space.

## When Do I Stop?

I recommend that you do the full program for six weeks. Studies have shown that this is a sufficient amount of time for you to see good, measurable gains in hand function - and a significant decrease in pain levels. If your hand feels great after six weeks, and you feel like you're where you want to be, I recommend doing the range of motion (ROM) exercises for reducing stiffness at least several times a week, the strengthening exercises as least once a week, and the hand coordination exercise at least once a week *to maintain* the progress you've made.

On the other hand, if you have good pain relief after doing the program for six weeks, but you're still not quite where you want to be, continue with the program until you either reach your goal, or no further progress is being made. And, if you have not seen a lick of progress after doing the program in the book for three months, then it is not a good solution for your hand osteoarthritis.

The pages that follow contain exercise sheets for six weeks of workouts. Make additional copies as needed.

# Week 1: Monday

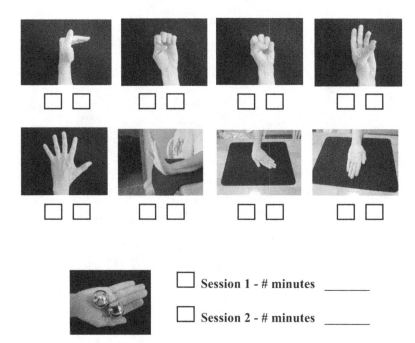

# lbs _____

# reps _____

# lbs _____

# reps _____

☐ rubber band?

# reps _____

☐ Session 1 - # minutes _____

☐ Session 2 - # minutes _____

# Week 1: Tuesday

☐ Session 1 - # minutes _____

☐ Session 2 - # minutes _____

# Week 1: Wednesday

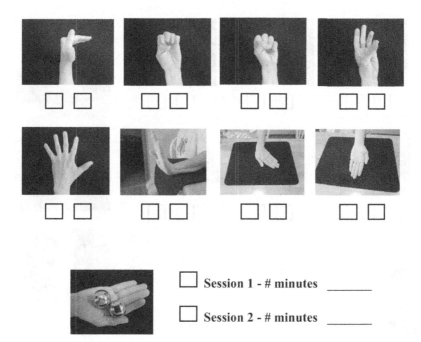

# lbs _____

# reps _____

# lbs _____

# reps _____

☐ rubber band?

# reps _____

☐ Session 1 - # minutes _____

☐ Session 2 - # minutes _____

# Week 1: Thursday

☐ Session 1 - # minutes _____

☐ Session 2 - # minutes _____

# Week 1: Friday

□ □   □ □   □ □   □ □

# lbs _____

# reps _____

□ □   □ □   □ □   □ □

# lbs _____

# reps _____

□ rubber band?

# reps _____

□ Session 1 - # minutes _____

□ Session 2 - # minutes _____

# Week 2: Monday

□ □   □ □   □ □   □ □

# lbs _____

# reps _____

□ □   □ □   □ □   □ □

# lbs _____

# reps _____

□ rubber band?

# reps _____

□ Session 1 - # minutes _____

□ Session 2 - # minutes _____

# Week 2: Tuesday

☐ ☐    ☐ ☐    ☐ ☐    ☐ ☐

☐ ☐    ☐ ☐    ☐ ☐    ☐ ☐

☐ Session 1 - # minutes _____

☐ Session 2 - # minutes _____

# Week 2: Wednesday

☐ ☐    ☐ ☐    ☐ ☐    ☐ ☐

☐ ☐    ☐ ☐    ☐ ☐    ☐ ☐

# lbs _____

# reps _____

# lbs _____

# reps _____

☐ rubber band?

# reps _____

☐ Session 1 - # minutes _____

☐ Session 2 - # minutes _____

# Week 2: Thursday

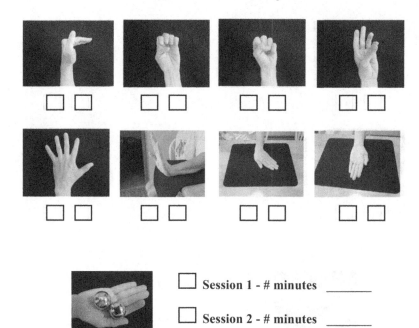

□ □  □ □  □ □  □ □

□ □  □ □  □ □  □ □

□ Session 1 - # minutes _____

□ Session 2 - # minutes _____

# Week 2: Friday

□ □  □ □  □ □  □ □

□ □  □ □  □ □  □ □

□ Session 1 - # minutes _____

□ Session 2 - # minutes _____

# lbs _____

# reps _____

# lbs _____

# reps _____

□ rubber band?

# reps _____

# Week 3: Monday

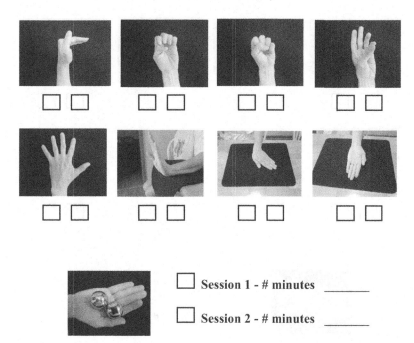

# lbs _____

# reps _____

# lbs _____

# reps _____

☐ □   ☐ □   ☐ □   ☐ □

☐ □   ☐ □   ☐ □   ☐ □

☐ rubber band?

# reps _____

☐ Session 1 - # minutes _____

☐ Session 2 - # minutes _____

# Week 3: Tuesday

☐ □   ☐ □   ☐ □   ☐ □

☐ □   ☐ □   ☐ □   ☐ □

☐ Session 1 - # minutes _____

☐ Session 2 - # minutes _____

# Week 3: Wednesday

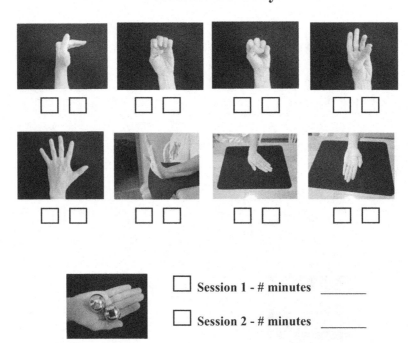

# lbs _____

# reps _____

# lbs _____

# reps _____

☐ rubber band?

# reps _____

☐ Session 1 - # minutes _____

☐ Session 2 - # minutes _____

# Week 3: Thursday

☐ Session 1 - # minutes _____

☐ Session 2 - # minutes _____

# Week 3: Friday

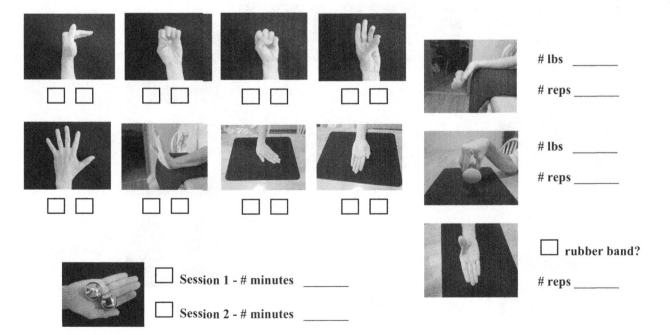

□ □    □ □    □ □    □ □

# lbs _____
# reps _____

□ □    □ □    □ □    □ □

# lbs _____
# reps _____

□ rubber band?

# reps _____

□ Session 1 - # minutes _____
□ Session 2 - # minutes _____

# Week 4: Monday

□ □    □ □    □ □    □ □

# lbs _____
# reps _____

□ □    □ □    □ □    □ □

# lbs _____
# reps _____

□ rubber band?

# reps _____

□ Session 1 - # minutes _____
□ Session 2 - # minutes _____

# Week 4: Tuesday

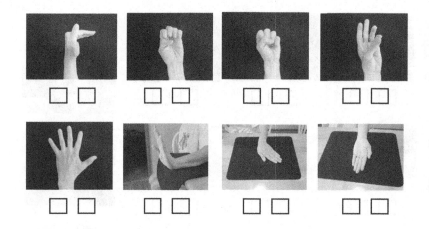

□ □    □ □    □ □    □ □

□ □    □ □    □ □    □ □

□ Session 1 - # minutes _____

□ Session 2 - # minutes _____

# Week 4: Wednesday

□ □    □ □    □ □    □ □      # lbs _____

# reps _____

□ □    □ □    □ □    □ □      # lbs _____

# reps _____

□ Session 1 - # minutes _____

□ Session 2 - # minutes _____

□ rubber band?

# reps _____

# Week 4: Thursday

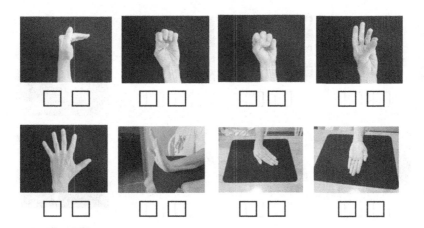

☐ ☐   ☐ ☐   ☐ ☐   ☐ ☐

☐ ☐   ☐ ☐   ☐ ☐   ☐ ☐

☐ Session 1 - # minutes _____

☐ Session 2 - # minutes _____

# Week 4: Friday

☐ ☐   ☐ ☐   ☐ ☐   ☐ ☐

# lbs _____

# reps _____

☐ ☐   ☐ ☐   ☐ ☐   ☐ ☐

# lbs _____

# reps _____

☐ Session 1 - # minutes _____

☐ Session 2 - # minutes _____

☐ rubber band?

# reps _____

# Week 5: Monday

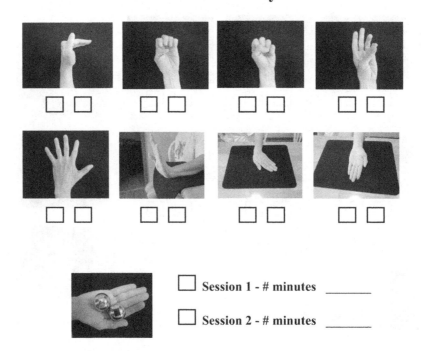

# lbs _____

# reps _____

# lbs _____

# reps _____

☐ Session 1 - # minutes _____

☐ Session 2 - # minutes _____

☐ rubber band?

# reps _____

# Week 5: Tuesday

☐ Session 1 - # minutes _____

☐ Session 2 - # minutes _____

# Week 5: Wednesday

□ □   □ □   □ □   □ □

# lbs _____

# reps _____

□ □   □ □   □ □   □ □

# lbs _____

# reps _____

□ rubber band?

# reps _____

□ Session 1 - # minutes _____

□ Session 2 - # minutes _____

# Week 5: Thursday

□ □   □ □   □ □   □ □

□ □   □ □   □ □   □ □

□ Session 1 - # minutes _____

□ Session 2 - # minutes _____

# Week 5: Friday

☐ ☐    ☐ ☐    ☐ ☐    ☐ ☐

# lbs _____

# reps _____

☐ ☐    ☐ ☐    ☐ ☐    ☐ ☐

# lbs _____

# reps _____

☐ rubber band?

# reps _____

☐ Session 1 - # minutes _____

☐ Session 2 - # minutes _____

# Week 6: Monday

☐ ☐    ☐ ☐    ☐ ☐    ☐ ☐

# lbs _____

# reps _____

☐ ☐    ☐ ☐    ☐ ☐    ☐ ☐

# lbs _____

# reps _____

☐ rubber band?

# reps _____

☐ Session 1 - # minutes _____

☐ Session 2 - # minutes _____

# Week 6: Tuesday

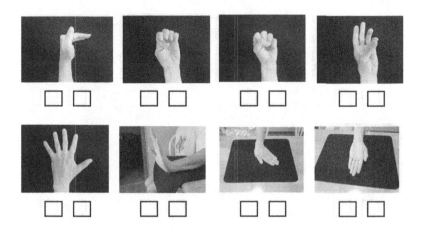

□ □  □ □  □ □  □ □

□ □  □ □  □ □  □ □

□ Session 1 - # minutes _____

□ Session 2 - # minutes _____

# Week 6: Wednesday

□ □  □ □  □ □  □ □

# lbs _____

# reps _____

□ □  □ □  □ □  □ □

# lbs _____

# reps _____

□ Session 1 - # minutes _____

□ Session 2 - # minutes _____

□ rubber band?

# reps _____

# Week 6: Thursday

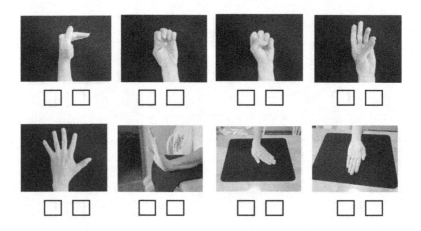

☐ ☐   ☐ ☐   ☐ ☐   ☐ ☐

☐ ☐   ☐ ☐   ☐ ☐   ☐ ☐

☐ Session 1 - # minutes _____

☐ Session 2 - # minutes _____

# Week 6: Friday

☐ ☐   ☐ ☐   ☐ ☐   ☐ ☐

# lbs _____

# reps _____

☐ ☐   ☐ ☐   ☐ ☐   ☐ ☐

# lbs _____

# reps _____

☐ rubber band?

# reps _____

☐ Session 1 - # minutes _____

☐ Session 2 - # minutes _____

# Why Measuring Your Progress Is *Very* Important

**O**kay. You've learned simple things you can do to help your hand osteoarthritis, started the exercises, and are on the road to recovery. So now what should you expect?

Well, we all know you should expect to get better. But what exactly does *better* mean? As a physical therapist treating patients, it means two distinct things to me:

- your hands start to *feel* better

  and

- your hands start to *work* better

And so, when a patient returns for a follow-up visit, I will re-assess them, looking for specific changes in their hand **pain**, as well as their hand **function**.

In this book, I'm going to recommend that readers do the same thing periodically. Why? Simply because people in pain can't always see the progress they're making. For instance, sometimes a person's hand pain doesn't seem to be getting any better, but they can move their hands better or do a few tasks that they couldn't do before - a sure sign that things *are* progressing. Or, sometimes a person still has significant hand pain, but they're not looking at the fact that it's actually occurring less frequently - yet another good indication that positive changes are taking place.

Whatever the case may be, if a person isn't looking at the big picture, and doesn't think they're getting any better, they're likely to get discouraged and stop doing their exercises altogether - even though they really might have been on the right track!

*On the other hand though*, what if you periodically check your progress and are keenly aware that your hand *is* making some changes for the better? What if you can *positively* see *objective* results? My guess is that you're going to be giving yourself a healthy dose of motivation to keep doing the exercises.

Having said that, I'm going to show you exactly what to check for from time-to-time so that you can monitor all the changes that are taking place. I call them "outcomes" and there are two of them.

## Outcome #1:
## Look for Changes in Your Pain

First of all, you should look for changes in your pain. I know this may sound silly, but sometimes it's my job to get a person to see that their pain *is* actually improving. You see, a lot of people come to physical therapy thinking they're going to be pain-free right away. Then, when they're not instantly better and still having pain, they often start to worry and become discouraged. Truth is, I have yet to put a patient on an exercise program for hand osteoarthritis and have them get instantly better. Better yes, but not *instantly* better.

Over the years, I have found that patients usually respond to the exercises in a quite predictable pattern. One of three things will almost always occur as patients begin to turn the corner and get better:

- your hand pain will be just as intense as always,
  however now it is occurring much less frequently

  or

- your hand pain is now *less* intense, even though
  it is still occurring just as frequently

  or

- you start to notice less intense hand pain *and* it is
  now occurring less frequently

The point here is to make sure that you keep a sharp eye out for any of these three changes as you progress with the exercises. If *any* of them occur, it will be a sure sign that the exercises are helping and you're on the right track. You can then look forward to the pain gradually getting better, usually over the weeks to come.

## Outcome #2:
## Look for Changes in Hand Function

Looking at how well your hand works is very important because many times hand function improves *before* the pain does. For example, sometimes a patient will do the exercises for a while, and although their hands will still hurt a lot, they are able to do many things that they hadn't been able to in a while - a really good indicator that changes are taking place *and* that the pain should be easing up soon.

While measuring your hand function may sound like a pain in the butt, it doesn't have to be. In this book, I'm recommending that readers use a quick and easy assessment tool known as the *Cochin Hand Functional Disability Scale* (Duruoz 1996).

While it may have a long name, this hand scale is actually a short and useful tool you can use to keep track of how well your hand is *functioning*. Studies show that it is a valid test (Poole 2010), has good test-retest reliability (Poole 2010), and is responsive to clinical changes (Poiraudeau 2001). And best of all, *it takes only a couple of minutes to complete*. Now that's my kinda test!

So what exactly does taking the scale involve? Not much.

- there are six possible answers to each question – each answer has a score of 0 to 6 points

- answer the 18 questions. For example, question one, "Can you hold a bowl" – if you can hold a bowl with *some* difficulty you'd put a "2" in the space provided – which gives you two points

- next, just add up the points to get your total score

On the next page is the scale, let's have a look…

*The Cochin Hand Functional Disability Scale*

Answers to the questions:
0=Yes, without difficulty
1=Yes, with a little difficulty
2=Yes, with some difficulty
3=Yes, with much difficulty
4=Nearly impossible to do
5=impossible to do

**In the kitchen**
1. Can you hold a bowl? __
2. Can you seize a full bottle and raise it? __
3. Can you hold a plate full of food? __
4. Can you pour liquid from a bottle into a glass? __
5. Can you unscrew the lid from a jar opened before? __
6. Can you cut meat with a knife? __
7. Can you prick things well with a fork? __
8. Can you peel fruit? __

**Dressing**
9. Can you button your shirt? __
10. Can you open and close a zipper? __

**Hygiene**
11. Can you sqeeze a new tube of toothpaste? __
12. Can you hold a toothbrush efficiently? __

**At the office**
13. Can you write a short sentence with an ordinary pen? __
14. Can you write a letter with an ordinary pen? __

**Other**
15. Can you turn a round door knob? __
16. Can you cut a piece of paper with scissors? __
17. Can you pick up coins from a table top? __
18. Can you turn a key in a lock? __

**Total score**_____

So what was your score? Keep in mind that scores will range anywhere from a 0 to a 90. Higher scores mean you're in bad shape, so your goal is to score as *low* as possible. In other words, a score of 0 means you're having *no* difficulty doing any of the activities listed on the scale, while a score of 90 means you're having a lot of trouble.

If you did score high though, don't worry. Just keep taking the scale every few weeks, and as you progress with the exercises, you should see your score go lower and lower as time passes. Remember, sometimes hand function gets better *before* the pain does.

---

### *Remember...*

✓ being aware of your progress is an important part of treating your hand osteoarthritis - it motivates you to keep doing the exercises.

✓ look for the pain to become less *intense*, less *frequent*, or both to let you know that the exercises are helping

✓ sometimes your hand starts to work better *before* it starts to feel better. Taking the *Cochin Hand Functional Disability Scale* from time-to-time makes you aware of improving hand function.

---

 # Comprehensive List of Supporting References

**W**ell, we've come a long way since page one. Now that we're at the end, I'd like to take a few minutes to show you all the research that went into this book.

The following is a list of all the randomized controlled trials and scientific studies that have been published in peer-reviewed journals that this book is based on. To make a long story short, there's no nonsense going on here - *every* piece of information you've just read has a good evidence-based reason for being here!

Having said that, I've included this handy reference section so that readers can check out the information for themselves if they wish.

## Chapter 1

Bagge E, et al. Osteoarthritis in the elderly: clinical and radiological findings in 79 and 85 year olds. *Annals of Rheumatic Diseases* 1991;50:535-539.

Bijsterbosch J, et al. Clinical and radiographic disease course of hand osteoarthritis and determinants of outcome after 6 years. *Ann Rhem Dis* 2011;70:68-73.

Harris P, et al. The progression of radiological hand osteoarthritis over ten years: a clinical follow-up study. *Osteoarthritis and Cartilage* 1994;2:247-252.

Zhang Y, et al. Prevalence of symptomatic hand osteoarthritis and its impact on functional status among the elderly. *Am J Epidemiology* 2002;156:1021-1027.

# Chapter 3

Garfinkel M, et al. Evaluation of a yoga based regimen for treatment of osteoarthritis of the hands. *J Rheumatology* 1994;21:2341-3.

# Chapter 4

Doerschuk S, et al. Histopathology of the palmar beak ligament in trapeziometacarpal osteoarthritis. *Journal of Hand Surgery* 1999;24A:496-504.

Lefler C, et al. Exercise in the treatment of osteoarthritis in the hands of the elderly. *Clinical Kinesiology* 2004;58:13-17.

Rogers M, et al. Exercise and hand osteoarthritis symptomatology: a controlled crossover trial. *Journal of Hand Therapy* 2009;22:10-18.

Pellegrini V. Osteoarthritis of the trapeziometacarpal joint: the pathophysiology of articular cartilage degeneration. I Anatomy and pathology of the aging joint. *Journal of Hand Surgery* 1991;16A:967-74.

Van Oudenaarde E, et al. Differences and similarities in electrical muscle activity for the abductor pollicis longus muscle divisions. *J Electromyogr Kinesiol* 1995;5:57-64.

Van Oudenaarde E. The function of the abductor pollicis longus muscle as a joint stabiliser. *Journal of Hand Surgery (Br)* 1991;16B:420-423.

# Chapter 5

Ranganathan V, et al. Skilled finger movement exercise improves hand function. *Journal of Gerontology: Medical Sciences* 2001;56A:M518-M522.

## Chapter 6

Boustedt C, et al. Effects of a hand-joint protection programme with an addition of splinting and exercise. One year follow-up. *Clin Rheumatol* 2009;28:793-799.

Stamm T, et al. Joint protection and home hand exercises improve hand function in patients with hand osteoarthritis: a randomized controlled trial. *Arthritis Care and Research* 2002;47:44-49.

## Chapter 7

Buurke JH, et al. Usability of thenar eminence orthoses: report of a comparative study. *Clinical Rehabilitation* 1999;13:288-294.

Carreira A, et al. Assessment of the effectiveness of a functional splint for osteoarthritis of the trapeziometacarpal joint of the dominant hand: a randomized controlled study. *J Rehabil Med* 2010;42:469-474.

Ikeda M, et al. Custom-made splint treatment for osteoarthritis of the distal interphalangeal joints. *Journal of Hand Surgery* 2010;35A:589-593.

Rannou F, et al. Splint for base-of-thumb osteoarthritis. A randomized trial. *Ann Intern Med* 2009;150:661-669.

Weiss S, et al. Splinting the degenerative basal joint: custom-made or prefabricated neoprene? *Journal of Hand Therapy* 2004;17:401-406.

## Chapter 9

Duruoz M, et al. Development and validation of a rheumatoid hand functional disability scale that assesses functional handicap. *J Rheumatol* 1996;23:1167-72.

Poiraudeau S, et al. Reliability, validity, and sensitivity to change of the Cochin hand functional disability scale in hand osteoarthritis. *Osteoarthritis and Cartilage* 2001;9:570-577.

Poole J, et al. Self-reports and performance-based tests of hand function in persons with osteoarthritis. *Physical and Occupational Therapy in Geriatrics* 2010;28:249-258.

Made in the USA
Coppell, TX
24 September 2023

21977803R00057